CRACKING THE
WEIGHT LOSS CODE
FOR WOMEN

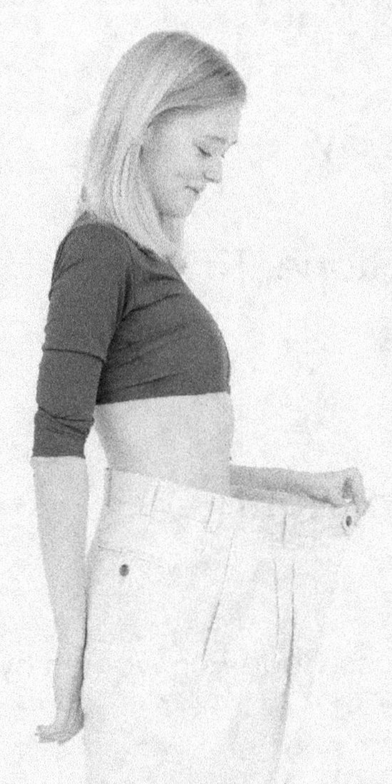

HEALTHY WAYS TO
LOSE 48 POUNDS
IN 112 DAYS

JAMIE STONE, RDN

Cracking The Weight Loss Code For Women

Healthy Ways To Lose 48 Pounds In 112 Days.

By

Jamie Stone, RDN

Copyright

Cracking The Weight Loss Code For Women by Jamie Stone, RDN

Legal Disclaimer

The Information contained in this book is the opinion of the author and is based on the author's personal experiences and observations. The author does not assume any liability whatsoever for the use of or inability to use any or all the information contained in this book, and accepts no responsibility for any loss or damages of any kind that may be incurred by the reader as a result of actions arising from the use of information found in this book. Use this information at your own risk.

The author reserves the right to make any changes he deems necessary to future versions of the publication to ensure its accuracy.

TABLE OF CONTENTS

Cracking The Weight Loss Code For Women

Healthy Way To Lose 48 Pounds In 112 Days.

Copyright

TABLE OF CONTENTS

Introduction: The basics

Before we begin, a few critical points must be addressed. Weight loss is a mental game. You will alter your physique if you change your thinking. It's unavoidable.

When we say "change your mind," we don't mean go from nibbling cookies to devouring cake. What we're discussing here is the attitude that underpins all weight loss. The basics are the same regardless of your age or gender.

First and foremost, you must quit disliking your body. Far too many women have terrible self-images. They believe they are overweight and unattractive in comparison to the other ladies. You may have desired the 'thigh gap,' but The Gap does not even carry your size.

"Why can't I look like her?"... "It sucks being me!"... "I have horrible fatty genes!"

These are just a few ways women punish themselves.

Here's the truth.

You need to love yourself for what you are. Flab, rolls, cellulite, and all. You need to start this weight loss journey from a place of self-love.

If you don't change this mindset, you will still have negative self-image issues even when you lose weight. You will never be good enough for yourself. Accept yourself, and from there, you can improve. This is a journey and not an overnight miracle.

Look in the mirror. That's your competition. Not anyone else.

You also need to understand that you CANNOT lose weight, by assuming that you have 'fat genes' or that it's more difficult for you to lose weight, you make it a self-fulfilling prophecy.

There will be times when you slip up. This is inevitable and par for the course. When pursuing any worthy goal, the journey is never linear.

It's often fraught with little setbacks, slip-ups, mistakes, etc. What you need to understand is that every setback is a setup for a comeback.
During those times when you slip up on your diet, don't throw in the towel and give up just because you made one mistake in your diet. If you eat a

slice of cake after work, don't blame yourself and go crazy the rest of the day by eating whatever else comes your way. Acknowledge your mistake and strive not to make any more.

If you are on track for the next few days, this one small slip-up will be negligible. If you throw your diet out of the window and give up, you can rest assured that the weight will pile back on.
You are not your mistake. acknowledge, correct it, avoid future mistakes and keep moving forward.
That is the only way to succeed.

Losing weight revolves around various essential aspects, including restoring and improving one's health, staying on track to achieve all your weight loss goals, and transforming and keeping a leaner body. To achieve successful weight loss, you must keep the weight loss basic principles in mind.
These include the following:

- Lose fat
- Stay motivated
- Gain muscle

In order to succeed, you have to take note that you need to make an extra effort, as there's no shortcut to shedding those unwanted pounds of yours.

Lose Fat: Diets Can Help You

Eating a correct and healthy balanced diet is essential when losing weight. Choose and follow a diet rich in fiber and protein and low in refined carbohydrates.
Once you have increased your fiber and protein intake, you will lose weight gradually, and your strong muscles will develop. Also, if you consume less refined carbohydrates, you get rid of piling calories, which don't provide the needed nutrients for your body.

Gain Muscles: Do Some Workouts

When losing weight, gaining muscle can help. It is because the fat will be burned to provide you with the right energy muscles require to stay alive. It's interesting to note that a pound of fat requires only three calories, while a pound of muscle needs 75-150
calories every day to work. Therefore, if you want to see results when losing weight, it's imperative that you do workouts.
You can consider any exercises or workouts. But, anaerobic and aerobic exercises are essential for your body to work harder. For better results, alter

your exercise routines to maintain the stimulation of your body.

Some consider weight loss programs just to do workouts. There are even others who enroll in a gym class. You don't need to spend a considerable amount of money when doing workouts. You can do workouts at your home. Just choose those exercises that will not require gym equipment. When doing workouts, take it seriously and stick to your plan. Learn to be motivated. Exercising regularly with consistency and commitment is a must. Do not make mistakes and expect quick results like most people do. You have to take note that it also takes
time to see results.

Staying Motivated

It is vital to accept that weight loss does not happen quickly. Losing weight is a journey in which you need to monitor your progress. With this, you will be able to see results while being motivated with your plan.
Losing weight may be easy for some because of using magic pills. But, if you want to improve your overall health and maintain a healthy weight, then

stay motivated and get going as this can make a difference.

1. Nobody Wakes Up 20 Pounds Heavier Overnight: Same As Losing Weight, It Is A Process

This is what the weight loss companies and diet pills manufacturers don't want you to know. Weight loss is a difficult process.

The concept is brain-dead simple. All you need to do is burn more calories than you consume. That's all it is. If you remove all the fluff and hype, it always boils down to this one principle.

You need to eat the right foods in the right quantities and get sufficient exercise.

The diet pill companies will tell you that you can achieve staggering results – "Lose 12 Pounds in 7 Days!" without starving yourself. Easy weight loss! That's always their angle. Common sense will tell you that these pills will never work. After all, how can you lose weight by eating something else?

To convince you that these pills work, the supplement companies will list a whole range of ingredients that sound exotic and supposedly have fat-burning properties.

Women believe this hype because the truth is a bitter pill to swallow. Cleaning up your diet and exercising is difficult. Taking weight loss pills is easy. And everybody wants it easy.

Easy often leads to disappointment, regret, and a loss of time and money. This is a heavy price to pay because, most often, you'll never see any results. That's why you see women going from pill to pill. That's why new weight loss supplements keep hitting the market. When people realize it's not working, they try the next product and the next.

This vicious cycle just doesn't end.

You need to understand that in most cases, you gain weight gradually. Nobody wakes up 20 pounds heavier overnight. Your body got fatter over time.

To lose fat, it will take time. This book says that you'll transform your body in 112 days, and it will. If you do what it says. It doesn't make wild promises of losing 20 pounds in a

week. In best-case scenarios, you will lose 3 to 4 pounds a week. In 4 weeks, you'll lose about 12 pounds or maybe 8.
It all depends on your body. The more surplus weight you have, the more weight you'll lose. It's a

strange contradiction, but generally, fatter people lose weight faster.
The leaner you get, the more challenging it becomes. Whatever the case may be, 28 days is a good time frame to aim for. You will definitely see the difference.

There is a quote in the fitness industry.

"It takes four weeks for you to see your body changing.
It takes eight weeks for your friends and family.
It takes twelve weeks for the rest of the world."

KEEP GOING

This is very true. In 28 days, the transformation that you see will give you the motivation to keep going because you know that what you're doing works. Most people give up because they can't see results fast enough.

Usually, they've just not given themselves enough time. You'll need to plan your weight loss, and then you'll realize just how long it will take you to reach your goal. We'll be looking at this in the next chapter.

What's really important is keeping things real for you. If you're looking at an eight week stretch to reach your dream body, you'll not lose motivation and give up after two weeks because you have six more weeks to go.
You also will not believe the hype that the infomercials and supplements throw at you.
Your body works at its own pace. It's not affected by hype or fantasies. Weight loss is based on natural laws. You wear what you eat. You need to move more… and you need to stay the course. This is what transforms your body.

It doesn't sound glamorous or fun… but the truth seldom does.

Nevertheless, you can lose weight. You ALWAYS can. Now let's move on to the next chapter, where I show you just how long it'll take you to reach your desired weight.

2. Calorie Deficit: Planning & Tracking Your Progress

The first thing you need to do is to check what your daily caloric deficit should be.
You can go here and check that.

http://www.freedieting.com/tools/calorie_calculator.htm

Being at a daily caloric deficit is the most important factor that determines if you will succeed or fail.
You could eat clean, watch your diet and exercise daily… BUT… if you're at a caloric surplus, you will never see your weight drop.

This is the reason why so many people struggle to lose weight and never see progress.

So, what is a caloric deficit?

It simply means a deficiency in the number of calories consumed comparable to the number of calories required for the maintenance of current body weight.

In other words, you're consuming fewer calories than your body uses. Now your body has no other option but to tap into its fat stores for fuel.

This is the major way you will deplete your body's fat stores and lose weight. Ideally, it would be prime if you aimed for around a 500-calorie deficit daily. You don't need to obsess over the numbers and strive for perfection. As long as you're within the 400 to 600 range, you'll be just fine and lose weight steadily.

In order to know your calories, you can visit this site.

http://www.freedieting.com/tools/calorie_calculator.htm

All you need to do is fill out the necessary fields and click on the "calculate" button.

You'll now be shown three different numbers.

Maintenance means that if you consume this number of calories, your weight will neither go up nor go down.

Fat loss denotes a caloric deficit. This is the number that you need to aim for in order to lose weight.

Extreme Fat Loss is an indicator that you should not drop your calories below this number.
So, if you wish to lose 20 pounds and you're losing about 2 pounds a week, you'll be looking at a time frame of 10 weeks, that is about two and a half months.

It seems long, doesn't it?

Here's what Earl Nightingale once said – "Don't let the fear of the time it will take to achieve something stand in the plan of you doing it. The time will pass anyway; we might just as well put that passing time to the best possible use."

Even if it takes you 10 weeks, go for it.

Most women never see any results. This guide gives you results.

However, if you need 10 weeks, you're not going to achieve it in 28 days. If we follow the example mentioned above, you'll lose 8 pounds in 28 days. It may not look like much, but it is definitely going to be a visible difference. Your face will become slimmer. Your belly and thighs may shrink a little. You'll be amazed.
And that's the whole point of this book. To show you what's possible, and from there you keep going. If it takes you 10 weeks, you just keep doing what you've been doing these 28 days till you reach the ten weeks.

You must stay the course!

Success is nothing more than a few straightforward disciplines, practiced
every day.

Tracking Your Progress

What is measured becomes managed. As a result, it's critical that you track your progress and keep a tight check on your nutrition and workout.
The first step is to weigh oneself using a weighing scale. This should be done once a week on the same day and time.

Do not weigh oneself on a daily basis since your weight can vary, which may be discouraging. Once a week would be enough, and any weight decrease will be reflected.
Please keep in mind that the scale weight only offers you a broad notion and is not indicative of body composition.
For example, if you lose 3 pounds of fat while gaining 2 pounds of muscle, the scale will only indicate a 1 pound decrease. This can be quite deceiving. You'd really made terrific progress and would appear different since fat takes up much more area than muscle.

That is why you also need to take photos of your body once every 2 weeks. With photos, the difference in your appearance will be more evident and you'll feel more motivated.

Many people are much more amazed to see before and after photos instead of just a difference in numbers on a scale.
If possible, get your body fat percentage measured. You can ask your doctor to do this and he or she will probably use calipers to determine your body fat percentage.

This is an accurate measurement to go by and your goal will be to lower your bodyfat percentage to what's ideal for you.
Using a tape measure to record down the measurements of different parts of your body is helpful too. You can encircle the tape around the middle of your thigh, your arm, hips, chest, etc.

It's important that you measure the same places in future to keep things accurate. With time, you'll notice the inches dropping.
Even if the scales show no difference after 2 weeks of exercise, the tape measure will definitely show you if you have become smaller.
Muscle is a lot denser than fat and takes up much less space.

In the first 3 to 4 weeks, it may seem like the results are slow. Losing a few pounds here and there may make it all seem like a total waste of time. You must understand that there are changes happening in you.
The body is adapting. Your metabolic rate is increasing. The body is starting to tap into its fat stores for fuel. All this is happening on the inside but you do not see obvious

results on the outside. This discourages the majority of women who quit on their weight loss program within the first month.

Most give up after 2 weeks!

They take a break and go back to their poor eating habits and sedentary lifestyle. 2 months later they decide to lose weight again.

When does it ever end?

This is the biggest mistake. You've just turned on the ignition and before the pedal hits the metal, you've given up.

Motivation is what gets you started. Habit is what keeps you going.

When you embark on a weight loss journey, give yourself an end date 100 days later. Do not stop before you reach that 100 days or you reach your weight loss goal.
There may be occasions where you slip-up on your diet. There may be times when you skip your workouts. There may even be weeks where there is

no change in weight. Despite all these, keep going till you reach the 100-day mark.

If you hate starting over, stop giving up. Three months from now, you will thank yourself. Do not give up on yourself and kill off your weight loss dreams before they have time to bloom.
Most visible weight loss can be seen after 90 days. That's about 3 months. You absolutely must give yourself 3 months.
Track your progress weekly and if things don't seem to be changing for the better, tweak your workouts and diet.

This is the best way to lose weight without losing your way.

3. Understanding and Controlling Hunger : Overcoming Emotional Overeating

Let's be honest. You'll have to eat less if you want to lose weight. Yes... yes... You do not wish to. You like to eat. Do you really need to limit your calorie intake?

Yes.

What if you consume the same amount of food and only exercise? No. You should still eat less.

Ok... ok. You'll eat the same amount, exercise as much as you can, and take a few slimming pills as well. Is it all right? No. You will still need to eat less.

We may proceed now that we've established that fact. When we advise eating less, we don't imply you have to eat like a bird. There will always be enough food to keep you strong, fit, and healthy.

People nowadays overeat, which is a concern in society. They eat when they are content. They eat when they are depressed. They eat when they're hungry and when they're not... out of fear of being hungry later.

When you try to limit calories, you will undoubtedly eat less than you are used to. Because you're already in the habit of consuming a particular amount of food every day, your body will feel a little hungry.

This is typical. You are not hungry. Your body will need time to acclimate to the lower calorie intake. There will be some discomfort, and you may find yourself thinking about eating frequently. You must practice willpower and refrain from eating. Maintaining a calorie deficit is critical to reducing weight.
Consider it a challenge that you can overcome. Many women regard diet control as a tremendous pain in the buttocks.

This chapter contains seven techniques for controlling your hunger. These will help you curb your desires to some extent. Keep in mind that your hunger will naturally decrease after a week of sustaining a calorie deficit.

You'll want to eat less if you eat less. Your stomach will contract, and you will need less food to be satisfied.

That may take a week or two to happen. Depending on how much you've been eating daily; it may take longer but rest assured that you will need less food as you go along.

7 Tips For Curbing Hunger

1. Skip breakfast.

This runs contrary to everything you've heard so far. However, studies have shown that the later you have your first meal, the less you'll eat throughout the day. If you must have breakfast, go ahead, but keep it light and ensure it is protein based. "Skip" the sugary cereals and white bread.

2. Drink lots of water.

It'll make you feel full, and people often mistake thirst for hunger. It would help if you also were sufficiently hydrated to accelerate fat loss.

3. Consume a tablespoon or 2 of virgin coconut oil daily.

It has been shown to reduce one's appetite, make a person leaner and also less prone to storing fat.

4. Stay active throughout the day.

Sedentary activities such as vegetating in front of the TV for hours, playing video games non-stop, watching movies at the cinema, etc., will automatically make you want to pop something in your mouth to munch. Avoid these activities.

5. Eat lots of vegetables.

Vegetables such as broccoli, spinach, carrots, cauliflower, kale, celery, etc., contain a ton of beneficial properties. Not only are they good for your health, but they will also leave you feeling fuller for longer.

6. Use smaller plates.
This is a psychological trick. Smaller plates look fuller with less food. So, your brain automatically assumes you're eating a lot when you're not.

7. Go to bed earlier.

A bad habit that many people engage in is binge eating at night. This is usually because they're awake watching TV and end up feeling hungry. If you find that you're getting hungry at night, go to bed earlier. You will not struggle against cravings.

Follow the tips above and you will reduce the amount that you eat. Once you achieve this feat, your weight loss will go from being a possibility to a probability and, finally, a reality. Your diet is that important to your success. Never forget that.

4. Do You Need To Diet?

You don't need to diet... but you do have to stick to a diet plan.

Does that make sense?

Many women make the mistake of starving themselves in order to lose weight quickly. This is unhelpful and works against them.

You must be on a diet that is appropriate for you... and, most importantly, you must be in a calorie deficit.

You will lose weight as long as you are in a calorie deficit.
"What if I ate junk food and yet maintained a calorie deficit?" you're undoubtedly thinking.

Yes, in theory. It's not that straightforward... but yeah. You can lose weight even if you eat fast food, processed food, and junk food... whatever you want to call it. You are aware of these foods.

As stated in Chapter 1, if you consume fewer calories,

You will lose weight if you eat less than your maintenance amount.

Therefore, theoretically speaking, even if you were on a junk food diet the entire day but you were consuming about 500 calories less than your maintenance level, you will lose weight.

Many overweight or obese women, almost always have a very poor diet. It is extremely difficult for them to switch from a diet that is so high in processed/junk food to one that is clean and wholesome.

Expecting to change your diet overnight is a recipe for disaster. Due to failure, This must be done gradually and incrementally. As a result, your best line of action will be to continue eating. The way you've been doing it, but aim for a calorie deficit. That basically implies you'll be eating less junk stuff than you were accustomed to. This alone will assist you in losing weight.

However, while the aim is to reduce weight and get healthier, The ultimate objective should be to remove junk food from your diet and consume more nutritious foods.

Make one tiny good modification to your diet every week. If you often have two cheeseburgers at lunch, followed by a Coke. That may be replaced by a crispy tuna wrap and a glass of cold coconut water.

This is simple psychology. It's only one dinner. Continue until this becomes a habit, and you gradually but steadily replace all of the junk food with healthful but appetizing meals.

Healthy meals may also be delicious. You are not foregoing flavor or enjoyment by eating properly. It's just a matter of getting your taste buds and body to enjoy eating healthy foods. Over time this can be achieved.

Meanwhile, you can eat junk food and yet lose weight when on a calorie-restricted diet
You should also be aware that junk foods are low in nutrients. That means that you might be consuming junk food and after a short period of time are still hungry. This is because your body is lacking in nutrients it requires. This is one of the reasons why, if your diet is inadequate, you will constantly be overweight.

No matter what you eat, you will feel hungry. It is also worth noting that various bodily functions will stop you from losing weight after a certain point. The human body is a very complicated entity. Because you are on a calorie deficit, it will lose weight for a while. However, with time, you will find it increasingly difficult to do so.

It's not just a mathematical calculation where calories in must equal calories out.
Other considerations include the thermogenic impact of the calories ingested, the quality of the calories consumed, and so forth.

So, ideally, you can eat junk food while being calorically deficient. Wean yourself off them gradually over a month or two. Stop eating bad meals and start eating healthier.

Of course, you may eat junk food every now and again.
However, many people who have made the move never feel the same way again or want to consume junk food.

One of the best ways of eating to lose weight will be to consume foods that help with the fat burning process.

By including these foods in your diet, you'll not only feel more satiated but the body will burn more calories too. Unlike weight loss supplements, these foods actually work and they're cheaper.

Foods That Help Burn Fat

- Almonds
- Eggs
- Olive Oil
- Green Vegetables
- Oatmeal
- Berries
- Lean meat & Oily fish
- All natural Peanut butter
- Green Tea
- Legumes & Beans
- Avocadoes

Just by consuming these foods, you'll be able to curb your hunger and also hasten the fat-burning process.
So, while you do not need to follow a highly restricted diet and starve yourself; you should aim to consume foods that are beneficial to your health.

You'll be amazed at how much good food you can eat when it's not processed. In the next chapter, we'll look at what the best foods are for you and what is the best thing you can do to lose weight.

5. Whole Foods and Wrong Foods : Guide Your Gut

Before telling you what the good foods to eat are, here is one of the BEST ways to lose weight fast.

Are you ready?

Cut Your Carbohydrate Intake and Processed Foods!

Carbohydrate intake is one of the biggest factors affecting the speed at which you lose weight. In fact, the main reason most women gain weight is because they consume too much-processed carbs.

When you eat processed carbs such as donuts, pasta, white bread, white potatoes, etc., the calories quickly add up, and the body has a lot of fuel.
It shuttles all the excess fuel into its fat stores, and that's how you gain weight. Furthermore, processed carbs usually cause a spike in insulin levels which indirectly leads to weight gain. A double whammy.

There is no doubt that limiting your carb consumption can help you lose weight. In fact, research has shown that limiting your carbohydrate intake is more beneficial than limiting your calorie intake.

Therefore, you will lose considerably more weight in the same amount of time if you are on a 500-calorie deficit per day and have a low-carb consumption as opposed to if you were eating carbs while on a deficit.

If so, does it make sense? Simply said, fewer carbohydrates result in greater fat reduction. Nice, huh? Of course!

Your body will burn more fat from your fat reserves when you eat fewer carbohydrates since there are fewer carbohydrates available for your body to use as fuel. Thus, fat loss is quickened.

Your body will have lower blood sugar levels, and those with diabetes will see an improvement in their condition. A low-carb diet also prevents type 2 diabetes because it improves your body's insulin sensitivity.

Your levels of good cholesterol will rise, while those of bad cholesterol will decline. Many individuals believe that eating fat will raise your cholesterol. The truth is that a high carb intake also has an adverse impact on your cholesterol levels. This runs contrary to popular belief yet studies show that a low-carb diet has more positive effects on your triglycerides than a low-fat diet.

It is important to note that you should never take things to extremes. This applies to carb restriction too.

There are diets such as the Atkins diet which is based on severe restriction of carbs for long periods of time. This is detrimental to your body because you will end up fatigued, moody and weak.

The diet is not sustainable and once you come off it, you will gain whatever weight you lost and a bit more.

Excessive carb restriction will compromise your immune system, lead to muscle loss, slow down your fat burning and put you in a weight loss plateau.

Your body's testosterone production will fall and you will have a suppressed thyroid output. You'll also develop leptin resistance which doesn't bode well for fat loss.
So, what do you do? How do you strike the right balance? You want the best of both worlds, don't you?

This can only be accomplished with a method known as carb cycling. You'll abstain from them for periods of three to six days.

Aim for 5 to 6 days of very little or no carbohydrates if you are overweight or obese and have poor metabolism.
You need to restrict your carb intake for 3 to 4 days if you only need to shed a few more pounds.
You will have one day of carbohydrate consumption after the time of carb restriction. You should "refeed" on this day.
If you eat enough carbohydrates on this day, you will provide your body with the fuel it requires. As your body's fuel reserves are refilled, your metabolism will increase, and you'll feel more energized.

Avoid sugary carbohydrates and choose whole-grain pasta, bread, and sweet potatoes instead. An extra 500–700 calories beyond the maintenance level should be your goal. This will restart your body's fat-burning process.

Use this technique repeatedly to accelerate your fat loss and improve your health. The day will come when you won't crave for carbs or processed junk foods.

When your body becomes healthy, its tastes will change. That's why fit people are constantly able to make wise food choices.

Once you have gotten over the hump of ditching these foods, the rest is easy.

Your insulin sensitivity will improve, the pounds will drop and you will look and feel like a brand new you.

There is a saying – "Your abs are made in the kitchen, not the gym." What that means is that almost 80% of your success at weight loss or getting lean is dependent on your diet.

When it comes to weight loss, the majority of your attention must be given to your diet.

The 7 foods listed below will sabotage your weight loss efforts.

There is absolutely no doubt that you have everything to gain and nothing to lose by giving these foods a pass.

The problem is that many people love these comfort foods and hate giving them up. Sugar is addictive.

The more sugary foods you eat, the more you'll crave. So, by eliminating them slowly, you'll slowly condition your body to crave for these foods less and less.

7 Foods You Should AVOID at All Costs!

- Doughnuts are probably one of the unhealthiest foods on the planet. They consist of nothing more than refined carbohydrates and sugar.

They are high in calories, fats, carbs and other preservatives.

Continued consumption of doughnuts will lead to weight gain and digestive problems.

- Fast food. Enough said.

- Chips are just about everybody's guilty pleasure. Ah… the joys of crunching on them while watching a movie. Chips have high levels of trans fats due to the hydrogenated vegetable oils that are used to fry the chips. This will lead to weight gain and cardiovascular disease.

- French fries. It has been said that French fries are more deadly than cigarettes. There may be some truth in this. High in trans fats and carcinogens, these foods can cause cancer.

- Bagels are another crowd pleaser. It has a very high glycemic index. It causes insulin spikes that create inflammation in the body along with other health issues. Acne, body aches, clogged arteries, mood swings, etc. are all side effects of unstable insulin levels… and of course, weight gain.Skip the morning bagel. It's better to skip the bagel than go for a 30 minute walk. That roughly gives you an idea of how detrimental it is.

- Microwaved popcorn. All the rage these days. Convenient, tasty and fun. Yet, they contain carcinogens and diacetyl. Both cause cancer.

- Cereals are another fat gain culprit. Most cereals are not good for your body despite being marketed as "healthy natural foods". There is hardly anything natural about cereals. They are genetically modified foods that can harm you in the long run.

Just avoiding unhealthy foods is half the battle won. Always remember the long term effects. Don't give in to sinful pleasures in the short term which may lead to suffering in the long run.

Essential Foods to Consume

Proteins

Compared to carbohydrates or lipids, protein digestion uses more energy. Therefore, if you consume a piece of beef with roughly 200 calories, you may theoretically expend 40 calories in the process of digestion. Ice cream, on the other hand, requires extremely few calories to digest.

This means that a significant portion of your daily calories should come from meals high in protein. Legumes and meat are fantastic providers of protein. If you are following a weight training regimen, the protein will also aid in your muscular growth. 0.8 grams per pound of body weight is a good target.

The protein will increase muscular growth. You end up burning more fat when you have greater muscle. Being in this cycle is beneficial. You may have noticed that folks who are physically active and muscular can get away with consuming more. All the time, their muscles burn more calories.

Skinless chicken, lean beef, tuna, sardines, chickpeas, eggs, and salmon are all excellent sources of protein. Omega-3 fatty acids are present in the fish. Because of this, the body may benefit from them much more.

The chemical properties in certain foods trigger off certain processes in the body that cause fat loss. So, eating these foods will make your body wake up and burn more fat.

Green Tea

Green tea is one of them. Do not use sugar. It may not taste great but it works.

Other Foods

Chilies, lemons, oranges, mangoes, garlic, ginger and onions are all foods that contain many powerful antioxidants and nutrients that strengthens your immune system. When you are strong, your workouts will be better and you will burn more fat.

One common problem most women face when they first embark on a weight loss program is that they constantly feel hungry.

Food is always on their mind and it takes a toll on their willpower.

One way to prevent this is to consume foods that are high in fiber and digest slowly. You will feel fuller for a longer period of time.

Fiber-rich foods digest swiftly and go through the digestive system more quickly. As a result, there is a lower likelihood of gaining weight since fewer calories are absorbed.
Eat things like brown rice, broccoli, whole-wheat bread, oatmeal, and oats. You should include broccoli frequently in your diet since it is very healthy for your body.

Consuming whole meals rather than processed ones is the main objective here. The entire foods are often located around the outside of most supermarkets.

You will be keeping yourself away from the processed foods as long as you stay away from the stuff in the inner aisles and shelves.
Last but not least, despite how healthy these foods are, you can only use them to reduce your weight if you follow a calorie deficit diet and a regular exercise routine.

A calorie deficit while following a healthy diet and an effective exercise regimen are the two essential elements of any fat reduction program. The rest is simply icing on the cake.

As a result, regardless of how healthy and clean your food is, make sure you continue to have a daily calorie deficit.

Water Not Wine

While there is nothing wrong in drinking the occasional glass of wine, when you're trying to lose weight, almost all the fluid you consume should only be water.

The easiest way to get fat is to drink your calories. Avoid sodas, commercially sold fruit juices, sports drinks, etc. You only need water!

And you should drink lots of it.

This is why you should drink water.

- Drinking ice-cold water in the morning speeds up your metabolism.
- It reduces your appetite. Any time you feel like snacking, drink a glass or two of water, and you'll feel full and be less likely to snack.
- It keeps you hydrated and healthy.
- Your body needs water to metabolize fat. It's part of the fat burning process.
- You'll be less likely to get dehydrated during exercise if you drink water regularly.

There's really no need to emphasize this any further. Drink enough water daily

6. The Power of Protein

One of the most effective methods for accelerating weight reduction is this one.

You will lose weight more quickly the more protein you eat. Protein digestion requires the body to expend extra energy. Proteins burn more calories than fats and carbohydrates, which take longer to digest.

Don't ever eat carbohydrates without protein. Never eat fat by itself without protein.

You may avoid an insulin increase only by eating these meals containing protein.

Eating eggs is one of the best methods to add protein to your diet.
One of the world's healthiest foods is an egg.

You should eat at least 3 eggs a day.

They have a negative reputation due to incorrect information concerning high cholesterol and other health issues.

This is quite ironic because while unhealthy cereals are promoted as being nutritious, eggs, which are healthy and beneficial, are demonized.

This book will clarify and set the record straight. The egg is a great source of protein, omega-3 fatty acids, and many other healthy nutrients.

Saturated and trans fats are what causes cholesterol in the body and not dietary cholesterol.

That implies that eating eggs with the yolk is perfectly OK despite what you have been instructed. Since the yolk contains the majority of the nutrients, it is really healthier.
Eggs are a great source of heart-healthy omega-3 fatty acids and lean protein, but they also include a number of other vital minerals.

Eggs are regarded as the ideal meal as well. In addition to 7 grams of protein and vitamins B6, B12, choline, leucine, L-arginine, and folate, they also include vitamin D. Although many of these vitamins may be unfamiliar to you, the important thing is that they are what your body actually needs.

What truly matters is how you prepare the eggs and that you consume them in moderation. Do not fry eggs in saturated fat or in vegetable oils. Use coconut oil or olive oil. Fry them lightly or half-boil them.

The point to note is that when you are losing weight, you should mix 3 egg yolks, and the rest should be egg whites. This is assuming that you're having more than 3 eggs.

The reason for this is that egg yolks, though high in protein, are calorie dense. So, you want the benefits that eggs provide, but you do not want to add more calories to your diet.

If you're still on the hedge about this, Rochester Centre for Obesity in America conducted research that proved eating eggs for breakfast could limit daily calorie consumption by more than 400 calories. Isn't that fantastic?

One tip to always note is that if you are consuming eggs daily, you will be getting more than enough protein. It would be ideal to avoid protein shakes and other commercial protein products sold in your health stores. Ideally, we should be getting our proteins
from natural sources.

Also, try to get eggs that are organic. They will contain less omega-6 fats and more omega-3 fats.

<u>If you're a vegetarian and don't eat eggs.</u>

There are many vegetables that are high in protein too. You can eat those and achieve the same benefits.

20 High Protein Veggies

- Peas (Green)
- Mange Tout (Edible-Podded Peas, cooked)
- Sweet Corn (Yellow)
- Succotash (Corn And Limas, cooked)
- Sprouted Beans, Peas & Lentils (Soybean Sprouts)
- Lima Beans (Cooked)
- Kale
- Broccoli Raab (Cime di Rapa, cooked)
- Parsley
- Artichokes (Globe or French)
- Broccoli
- Baby Zucchini (Courgettes)
- Garden Cress
- Beet Greens (Cooked)
- Arugula (Rocket)
- Brussels Sprouts (Cooked)

- Spinach (Cooked)
- Mushrooms (White, cooked)
- Collard Greens
- Mustard Greens

7. Workouts: Structure Your Workouts

It is crucial to maintain a healthy exercise routine that not only improves your stamina but also tones and strengthens your body.

A fantastic technique to burn calories and drop pounds is through cardio.

Millions of women worldwide concentrate ONLY on cardio exercises. This is incorrect since strength training is also essential for losing weight.
Your body burns more calories when at rest the more lean muscle mass it has.

That essentially means you'll be a fat burning machine throughout the day.

The best way to structure your workout will be to have 3 cardio sessions a week and two resistance training sessions.

The Power of Fasted Cardio

Cardio is extremely effective when done on an empty stomach.

You may have heard that exercising on an empty stomach is great for weight loss.

However, the idea of a strenuous workout so soon after waking doesn't appeal to most people.

It need not be difficult, which is excellent news. In reality, it's preferable to keep things simple.

Going for a quick walk first thing in the morning is one of the finest strategies to lose weight. The ideal is a 20 to 30 minute stroll.

A dialogue should be possible while walking. You shouldn't be working so hard that you're gasping for air and panting.

Here, extreme intensity is not what we're going for.

Your body is fasting when you wake up in the morning. Your body would have digested the food, and your glycogen stores are low.

This implies that while you walk, your body will be compelled to burn fat for fuel. Your body uses its fat reserves as fuel during the 20 to 30 minutes that you walk.

This is a really effective technique that you may do every day because it isn't taxing.
Your metabolic rate will increase as a result of the morning walk, increasing your daily calorie expenditure.

If walking is not your thing, you may swim or ride a stationary bike instead.
Your body will burn fat when engaging in a cardiac exercise as long as the speed is modest, so your efforts will be rewarded.

Later in the day, you might want to do some strength training or a quick, high-intensity interval workout. That's good because the purpose of the early workout is just to accelerate the fat-burning process.

It's an extra method to assist you in achieving your weight goals more quickly. Anyone can use this strategy because it is so simple.

If a 10-minute stroll is the most you can muster, then do just that. You can gradually increase it to 20 or 30 minutes over time.

Really, there's no need to go longer than 30 minutes.

Give this method a try, and within a couple of weeks, you will see the difference.

Weight Training

Many women worry about getting bulky and muscular like men if they were to train with weights. This assumption is false.

Even men struggle with gaining muscle. Women who train with weights will look leaner and more defined, but they will not become manly.
You can cast aside all worries about looking like a female bodybuilder.

Bodyweight training such as squats, push-ups, lunges, dips and pull-ups are great ways to work your muscles and joints. It's crucial to work your muscles, or they will atrophy with age.

Look for exercises that tone your thighs, butt and arms.
These are common problem areas for many women. While cardio will help you shed the fat, strength training will give you the curves and

definitions that will make you look fit, healthy and radiant.

A short 10 to 15 minute full body workout done early in the day will work miracles. This type of workout is known as HIIT… High Intensity Interval Training.

Here's the kicker. You can even do a HIIT workout in one spot and still sweat like crazy.

For example, let's look at this workout circuit.

Sit Ups – 45 seconds

Burpees – 45 seconds

Jump Squats – 45 seconds

Push Ups – 45 seconds

High Knees – 45 seconds

Jumping Jacks – 45 seconds

Burpees – 45 seconds

Alternating Long Jumps – 45 seconds

Sit ups – 45 seconds

Push Ups – 45 seconds

Each exercise will have 15 seconds of rest before you move on to the next. You could do this workout in a cubicle. It takes up that little space…

BUT..

Most people will not be able to even make it to the 9th exercise.

Why?

Because of the intensity. You need to go as hard as you can go. There is no taking it easy. If all you have is 10 minutes, then it MUST be a hard 10 minutes.

The good news is that this is just 10 minutes. You'll be in the 'hurt box' during this time but you need to keep telling yourself…

"It's only 10 minutes! I can do this."

You could complete a workout within a commercial break. It's that fast. If you do this workout early in the day, your body will be in fat burning mode throughout the day because of the intensity.

It creates a situation in your body known as post-exercise oxygen consumption. That means your body will be burning calories at an accelerated rate for 10 to even 14 hours after your workout is over.

It's amazing what just 10 minutes can do.

The reason you do it early in the day is because your metabolism drops the moment you go to bed. By completing your training early in the day, you'll reap maximum rewards.

It's also worth noting that it's best that you make these short workouts full body workouts. Do compound movements such as squats, jumps, push ups, etc.,

By recruiting as many muscles in your body as you can, you'll be ensuring that your workout is engaging the whole body. Don't just try to wing it with simple exercises such as dumbbell curls and call it a day. All you have is 10 minutes. You have to make it count.

Even 3 of these short workouts a week will transform your body within a month. Go ahead and give them a try.

You will be amazed.

Do remember to have 2 rest days a week. You can split them up or you can have both days back to back. It's really up to you.

It is important to take a weekly break so that your muscles and central nervous system may rest. Going too hard without rest causes your body to get exhausted and agitated.

If you wind up reaching a weight loss plateau, you won't be able to lose weight again no matter what you do.

After that, you will need to rest for 4 to 5 days in order to recuperate. Your progress will be slowed down, and you could even put on weight.
Every week, take a two-day getaway.

Find the best resistance training and cardio exercises by doing some online research.

Challenge your body by mixing up your workouts. You'll quickly get leaner and stronger.

Add Fun To It

Make your exercise sessions fun. Find a workout buddy if you need one.

Don't repeat the same exercises each day. Even the most spirited lady can lose interest in monotony.

Try a novel approach. Kickboxing or yoga at the gym, perhaps. Attempt rock climbing as well!

Feeling like a dancer? See Shaun T's exercises and copy them.

Here, maintaining motion is essential. No matter what you do, your calorie deficit will lead to weight reduction.

The exercise is just intended to quicken the process.

Whatever you want, do it. Running, swimming, and bicycling.

What matters is that you MOVE daily. A sedentary
lifestyle is what causes obesity.

Keep moving and keep it fun.

8. Finding the Time

Most women are hard-pressed for time. You could
be the mother of a newly born child who needs your

full attention. Or you might be a career woman with demanding deadlines and you still need to juggle your duties as a wife.

We live in a fast paced world. Everybody is running the rat race to be the best rat. Time is a precious commodity that never seems to be enough. So what do you do?

You improvise. That's what you do.

To put things in perspective, you must realize that there are 24 hours in a day. A one hour workout is 4 percent of your day. A 15 minute workout is one percent of your day. An eight minute workout is "half a percent" of your day!

But what can I achieve in 8 minutes? A lot! Anybody, no matter how busy, can squeeze in 8 minutes. 8 minutes is too much? How about 6 minutes? What?! 6 Minutes?

Yes. 6 minutes of Tabata protocol.

Tabata Workout Instructions

The first six minutes of the novice workout are dedicated to warm-up. 2 minutes of warm-up time is divided into 2 sections of 30 seconds each. Exercise for one minute, followed by a two-minute cool-down.

1) Use a stationary bike, elliptical trainer, rowing machine, recumbent bike, versa climber, or other cardio machine that makes use of your legs' strong muscles and allows you to progressively increase the resistance, pace, etc.

The only alternative on a treadmill is to step onto the sides and stop completely since the machine won't react quickly enough to the necessary fast changes in velocity during a Tabata Protocol period because you need to relax for 10 seconds in between bouts of exercise.

2) Constantly monitor your heart rate. Keep track of your maximum heart rate during the whole workout and your recovery heart rate (see below)

3. Warm up at a slow speed for two minutes. To gradually raise your heart rate to a reasonable level, you may start off with low resistance and low RPMs (say 30-35 RPMs on a bike) for the first minute. Then, for the second minute, either increase the tension on your equipment one notch or gently increase the RPMs.

4) Begin by doing two intervals:
- First, if your feet are "flying off the pedals," crank up the tension one notch higher than where your warm-up finished.

- For 20 seconds, pedal (or go) at FULL SPEED, as quickly as you can, above 85 RPMs (if on a bike), even above 100 RPMs.

- For the following 10 seconds, pedal slowly. If you completed it correctly, you SHOULD notice a little increase in heart rate once you stop pedaling so quickly. This is a result of the oxygen debt you accrued, and it tells your body to supply your energy system with additional oxygen. Panting is a sign that your body is trying to obtain extra oxygen into your lungs so that it can power your energy system.

- Repeat once more (20 seconds all out fast, 10 seconds slow). Each time you enter the slow half of the interval, you should notice a slight increase in heart rate.

- Decrease the tension on your bike or other exercise equipment to 0 (the lowest setting) and cycle slowly for 2 minutes.

- Take your pulse or heart rate after your two-minute cool-down. Your recovery heart rate is shown here (RHR). Observe it. To determine when it is safe to increase intervals, you must compare your RHR from exercise to workout.

- Note the highest heart rate you were able to get while exercising. This might have happened in either your first or last interval (usually the last). It will PROBABLY exceed the maximum heart rate determined by subtracting your age from 220. If it isn't, that's alright; just be careful not to overdo it, especially when you're just starting out.

5) Perform this exercise three times each week; give yourself at least a full day between sessions to recover. Your body needs to mend itself, strengthen your heart and lungs, among other things.

6) Increase your fitness level gradually by starting with one interval and increasing it to eight intervals every time your RHR increases from your last session. When you notice an improvement in your RHR, you can then keep improving your cardio fitness by stepping up the tension or intensity.

You can read more about Tabata protocol on google to find out more. The point here is that you can cause a metabolic boost to your body and put it in fat burning mode within 6 minutes and you will be in a fat burning state for hours. Will it be easy? No. But it will be effective.

If you do not have time for one hour long workouts, do quick bursts of 15 minutes or even less. The difference is that the shorter workouts will have to be more intense.

However, it will be for a short while only.

There are also other methods to ensure that you burn more calories. Get yourself a pair of ankle weights and wear them throughout the day.

You will burn more calories when you walk and move. If you're a stay at home mom, get a haversack and add some weight in it. Throw in a telephone directory or 2 and wear the haversack.

The added weight will make everything more difficult and you will be burning more calories because of the added resistance.

Get yourself a Fitbit which will track the number of steps you take daily. Aim to increase the number of steps by 100 everyday.
Climb the stairs instead of using the elevator. Walk to the supermarket if you can.

If you're the mother of a newborn, get an infant sling and place your baby in it. Then proceed for a 30 minute walk. Excellent exercise for you and the baby gets a breath of fresh air too.

You may not have enough time. Yet, with a bit of imagination, you can incorporate many little practices and changes in your life to burn more calories. Once you have that done, get a journal and record your hourly activities.

See where your time goes. "Oh look! I'm watching Sex and the City reruns daily!"… ah hah! A time waster right there. Cut it out and spend that 30 minutes exercising. It will do you more good than watching Samantha, trying to get it on with all the guys in New York.

Do whatever you can with whatever time you have. Even if it's only 4 minutes.

9. Sleep Your Way To Weight Loss

Getting enough sleep is crucial to losing weight.

When you don't get enough sleep, your body is stressed out and releases a hormone called cortisol. This hormone leads to weight gain indirectly.

What most people fail to grasp is that being constantly deprived of sleep will take a toll on your health in the long run.

Research has shown that people who have less sleep eat more, feel hungrier and generally consume 350 calories more than required. Those who stay awake late often find themselves consuming snacks and heavy meals often.

Your body's insulin sensitivity and glucose tolerance levels will drop. This is bad since your body will go into fat-storage mode instead of being in fat-burning mode. When your insulin sensitivity is down, you will store fat much more easily. The same applies to glucose tolerance.

Lack of sleep also increases the body's stress hormone, cortisol.

Once again, the body's fat-burning ability decreases or, in a worst case scenario, just completely stops.

If you're eating on a caloric deficit and training daily, your body is already stressed out. It needs sleep to rest and repair itself. Not to mention de-stress.

There is a reason it is referred to as "beauty sleep".

All the best attempts at losing weight will be hampered if you can't afford to get enough sleep at night. Power naps during the day will not cut it.

You need to sleep at night for at least 7 hours. Most people claim to get by on less. They may… but at a price to their health in the long run.

Aim to be more productive so that you get more work done in the office and don't have to stay late. Stop watching late-night TV, and do not work out too close to bedtime.

Ideally, you should be working out during the day.

Try and meditate to free your mind from the daily stresses of life.

Remember, even if you win the rat race, you're still a rat. There is more to life than deadlines, targets and appraisals. Get enough sleep and you will find it much easier to shed the fat.

The power of a good night's sleep should never be underestimated.

Do ensure that you're getting at least 6 to 8 hours of sleep daily.

Don't burn the candle at both ends when you're on a weight loss journey.

10. Dealing with Slip Ups

It will happen. There is no doubt that it will take place sooner or later. "What's going to happen?" you ask.

It's inevitable that you will stray from your diet and eat something you know you shouldn't or you fail to work out when you know you should.

Almost everyone experiences it. Whether you succeed in your weight reduction efforts or abjectly fail depends entirely on how you respond to a mistake.

Let's start with discussing diet lapses. In order to establish a calorie deficit when losing weight, you often have to consume less than you normally would. Along with avoiding processed and junk food, you should concentrate on consuming wholesome, healthful meals.

However, the body is already accustomed to mindless eating, and you probably have a hidden addiction to processed and junk food. Many do, and when they try to stop eating these harmful foods, they experience cravings and mood swings.

The key point is to make the changes gradual. Only aim for a 500 calorie deficit daily.

This is a manageable amount, and you will not be feeling pangs of hunger.
You may feel a little peckish but it will be manageable. If you cut your calories too drastically, you will be feeling hungry all the time and this is sheer mental and physical torture.

Changing your foods overnight causes the same problem. Your body is not used to it.

Aim to gradually reduce consumption of bad foods and replace them with good ones.

If you drink 3 cans of soda daily, cut it down to 2 for a week and then bring it down to 1 can… and finally, put an end to the soda habit. Don't just give up sodas overnight.

Problems arise when people try to do too much too soon. They make things so challenging that compliance becomes a nightmare. People aim for perfection.

Sooner or later, they lose the battle of wills within themselves and give in to temptation and eat a greasy cheeseburger and fries or they polish off an entire bag of cookies.

When that happens, they feel guilty and think that they have failed. They then believe that they're destined to be fat, and they throw in the towel and give up on their goal. This happens to millions of people and is the reason why so many people quit.

The first point to note when you slip up is that you made a single mistake. You have not failed yet. You only fail when you give up. If you accidentally dropped your mobile phone, wouldn't you quickly pick it up, dust it off and keep it safely?

Surely you wouldn't keep dropping it and smashing it because of the first accident.

In the same way, acknowledge your slip-up and move on. Tell yourself that you will be more mindful of what you eat. Ease up on your stringent diet and allow flexibility while maintaining a caloric deficit. Do not deprive yourself of too much too soon.

As for your workouts, the same mindset should apply. If you miss a workout today, make sure you do one the next day. Never ever miss more than 3 workout sessions in a row, or you'll conveniently fall off track, and it will be very tough to go back.

If you dread exercising, you're either pushing yourself too hard or you're engaged in an activity that you have no interest in.

Exercise is intended to promote fat burning and raise metabolic rate. When it comes to losing weight, your food and calorie deficit are what actually count.

Diet errors and missed exercises are not the ends of the world, and your weight reduction goal should not come to an end as a result.

It is a journey, and it's inevitable that you get lost along the way every now and then. If you stay on track and keep going despite your setbacks, you will reach your goal. That's almost always how most people reach their goals. Hold fast to your chin and keep
moving forward.

11. Taking Time To Smell The Roses

There will be times when you just feel like giving up. This is normal.

What you need to do is relax and enjoy the process. Be satisfied with even a pound of weight loss. You can lose more the following week.

What matters is that you know that you'll get there, and you must stay positive.

Don't obsess over your weight. Maintain the caloric deficit, do your workouts, drink enough water, get enough sleep, make your workouts fun and relax.

You will reach your goal. Watch a movie or a comedy to destress. Go on a vacation but don't throw your diet away.

Always keep your chin up and keep going forward. Visualize where you want to be… and you'll get there.

Getting There and Staying There

Most women who lose weight often gain it back after a while.
Even people on TV shows such as The Biggest Loser gained all the fat they all once the show ended.

In order to stay slim, you need to change your lifestyle.
You'll need to practice whatever you're learned in this book for life.

Once you reach your ideal weight, you will need to consume your calories at maintenance level. This will ensure that you neither gain nor lose more weight.

Keep doing the workouts you're doing to stay fit.

You'll always have to be on the ball. A rolling stone gathers no moss… so you'll need to keep at it.

It took you so much effort to get to your weight loss goals… don't lose it all by going back to your old ways.

Eat healthy, stay active… and be happy.

Conclusion

Well… you've reached the end of the book.

If you follow what was stated in here without giving up, you will reach the body you desire.

Don't quit. If you're tired of starting over, stop giving up.

You can do it.

Millions of women have successfully lost weight and kept it off. If they can do it, so can you.

All the best in your weight loss journey.